Cambridge **Discovery Education**™

▶ **INTERACTI**

Series editor:

BONES
AND THE STORIES
THEY TELL

A2⁺

Diane Naughton

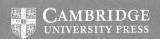

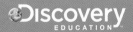

CAMBRIDGE UNIVERSITY PRESS
Cambridge, New York, Melbourne, Madrid, Cape Town,
Singapore, São Paulo, Delhi, Mexico City

Cambridge University Press
32 Avenue of the Americas, New York, NY 10013-2473, USA

www.cambridge.org
Information on this title: www.cambridge.org/9781107670549

First published 2014

Printed in Hong Kong, China, by Golden Cup Printing Company Limited

A catalog record for this publication is available from the British Library.

Library of Congress Cataloging-in-Publication Data

Naughton, Diane.
  Bones : and the stories they tell / Diane Naughton.
    pages cm. -- (Cambridge discovery interactive readers)
  ISBN 978-1-107-67054-9 (pbk. : alk. paper)
  1. Human skeleton--Juvenile literature. 2. English language--Textbooks for foreign speakers.
  3. Readers (Elementary) I. Title.

QM101.N38 2013
611'.71--dc23

                          2013025129

ISBN 978-1-107-67054-9

Additional resources for this publication at www.cambridge.org

Layout services, art direction, book design, and photo research: Q2ABillSMITH GROUP
Editorial services: Hyphen S.A.
Audio production: CityVox, New York
Video production: Q2ABillSMITH GROUP

Contents

Before You Read: Get Ready!

All people and most animals have bones. And bones can tell the people of today a lot about the past. Read on to find out how!

Words to Know

Look at the pictures. Then complete the definitions below with the correct words.

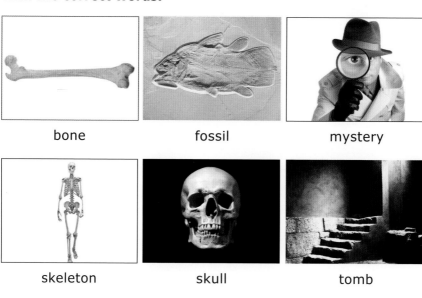

bone   fossil   mystery

skeleton   skull   tomb

1 _____ : something strange that we cannot explain
2 _____ : hard, white pieces in a person's head
3 _____ : a hard, white piece inside the body
4 _____ : a building for dead people
5 _____ : part of a plant or an animal that is kept inside rock for a long time
6 _____ : all the bones together inside the body

Words to Know

**Read the paragraph. Then complete the sentences below
with the correct highlighted words.**

Many years ago, Tiwanaku in Bolivia was a very important city
with many wonderful buildings. Now, we can see very little of these
buildings because people and nature have destroyed them. Today,
scientists are very interested in discovering the facts about Tiwanaku.
They go there and dig under the floor of the old buildings. They often
find things that were buried there thousands of years earlier. Sometimes
they find bones, and these bones can show us the secrets of life in
Tiwanaku.

1 I want to put a tree in the garden, so I'll have to
_____ a place for it.

2 Shh! Don't tell my _____ to anyone!

3 After my cat died, it was _____ under a tree in the
garden.

4 I had to find a new place to live when my house was
_____ in a fire.

5 I read lots of history books because I like _____
things about the past.

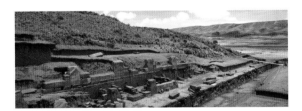

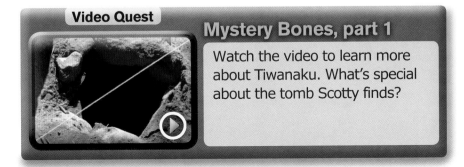

Video Quest

Mystery Bones, part 1

Watch the video to learn more
about Tiwanaku. What's special
about the tomb Scotty finds?

5

CHAPTER 1

Bones

WHAT DO YOU KNOW ABOUT BONES?

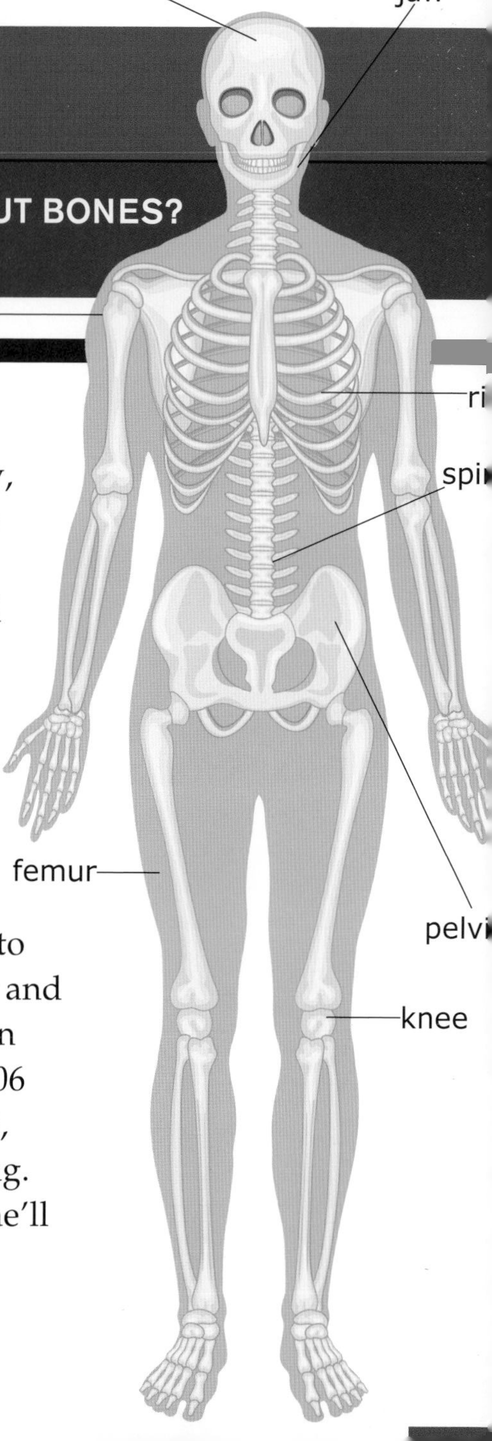

skull

jaw

shoulder

ri

spi

When you see bones in a museum, they look hard, dry, and dead. But when they are inside our bodies, they are living things. They grow and change, and they can even repair themselves when they are broken. Bones are amazing things!

When a **human** baby is born, it has about 270 soft bones. When the baby starts to grow, those bones get bigger and harder, and some of them join together. Adults have only 206 bones. By the age of about 25, a person's bones stop growing. Now the person is as tall as he'll ever be!

femur

pelvi

knee

One of the most important parts of the skeleton is the skull. The 22 skull bones are like a case for the brain. The smallest bone in the body is found here. It is called the stapes, and it is part of the ear. It is only 2.5–3.3 millimeters long.

The only skull bone people can move is the jaw. It is used to open, close, and move the mouth.

A person's spine goes down the middle of the back. It is very important because people need it to stand up straight. It also helps people move and bend.[1] The spine isn't one bone, but 26 small bones that look like the rings.

The ribs are connected to the spine. Most people have 24 ribs, 12 on the left and 12 on the right. Some people, however, are born with one or two ribs more or less. The ribs are like a case for the heart. So if someone falls, the ribs might get hurt, but the heart will be safe.

....

[1]**bend:** move your body so that it isn't straight

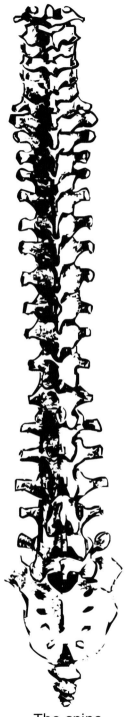

The spine

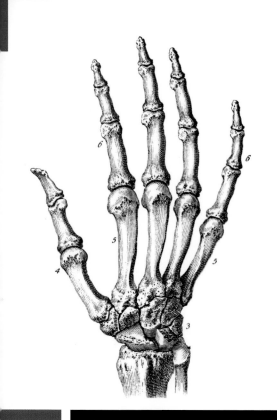
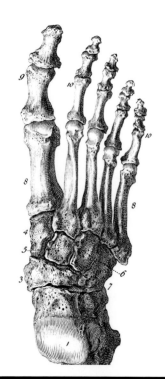

At the top of the leg is the femur. This is the longest, biggest, and strongest bone in the body. When people stand, walk, or run, all their **weight** falls on this bone.

More than 50 percent of a person's bones are in the hands and feet. There are 27 in each hand and 26 in each foot. This means we can move our hands and feet in many different ways.

Bones are very strong and very light. If a person **weighs** 100 kilograms, only about 15 kilograms of this is bone.

Video Quest

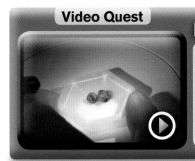

Mystery Bones, part 2

Watch the video to learn what the scientists discovered in the laboratory.[2] What does the corn[3] tell us?

But what happens to bones when people die? Well, sometimes bones are not destroyed for a long time, maybe for millions of years. Special scientists called paleontologists study old bones and teeth. They ask questions like these:

- Have all the skull bones joined together? (This tells them the person's age.)

- What are the teeth like? (This tells them about what the person ate.)

- How long is the femur? (This bone is about a quarter of a person's **height**, so they can guess how tall the person was.)

Bones can be the key to the secrets of history!

Paleontologists and other scientists learn things from bones.

....

[2]**laboratory:** a room where scientists work

[3]**corn:** a tall green and yellow plant that we eat

9

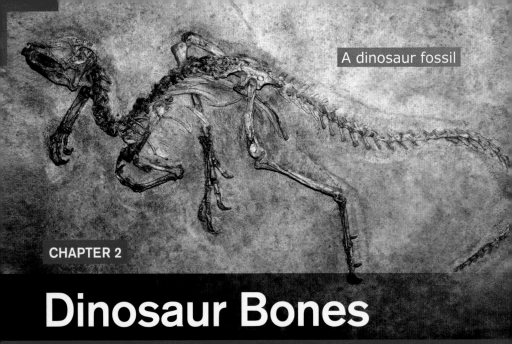

A dinosaur fossil

CHAPTER 2

Dinosaur Bones

WERE DINOSAURS BIG OR SMALL, FAST OR SLOW? DID THEY LIVE ALONE OR IN FAMILIES?

Today, dinosaurs are everywhere: but only in books, movies, and museums. Real dinosaurs lived in our world between 65 and 230 million years ago. That's about 62 million years before the earliest **humans**. So how do we know so much about them?

When an animal dies, the soft parts of its body are destroyed by nature. But sometimes the hard parts, like the skeleton and the teeth, are not destroyed. This happens when the animal's bones are covered quickly by rock. If the bones stay under this rock for a long time, they become fossils. And scientists can study fossils millions of years later!

The first dinosaur fossils were probably discovered thousands of years ago, but people didn't know what they were. The Chinese thought they were dragon bones, and they used them in medicine. And in England in 1676, an Oxford University teacher found a very big leg bone, but he believed it belonged to a giant.[4]

In 1841, the British scientist Richard Owen gave the name "dinosaur" to a group of animals. From his studies of bones, he showed that they all had the same kind of pelvis and straight legs (a bit like the human pelvis and legs today). He took the name from the Greek language: *deinos* meaning "terrible" and *sauros* meaning "lizard."

[4]**giant:** a very big person from stories

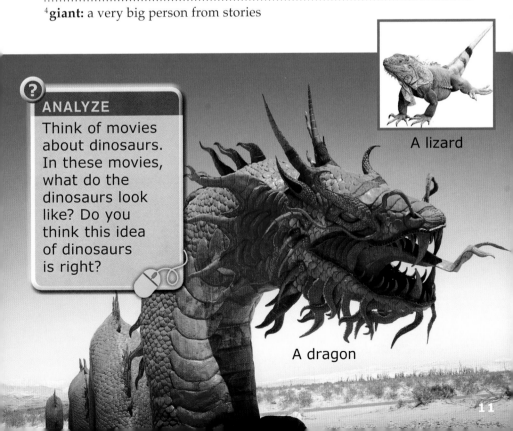

A lizard

ANALYZE

Think of movies about dinosaurs. In these movies, what do the dinosaurs look like? Do you think this idea of dinosaurs is right?

A dragon

11

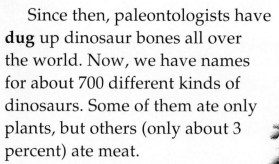

Since then, paleontologists have **dug** up dinosaur bones all over the world. Now, we have names for about 700 different kinds of dinosaurs. Some of them ate only plants, but others (only about 3 percent) ate meat.

Some dinosaurs were very, very big. The longest was *Seismosaurus*. It grew as long as 40 meters. And *Brachiosaurus* was the heaviest. At 80,000 kilograms, it weighed the same as 17 African elephants together. But other dinosaurs were very small. *Lesothosaurus* was only the size of a chicken.

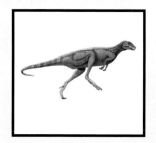

Seismosaurus was much longer than *Lesothosaurus*!

Some dinosaurs looked like birds and were very fast. *Dromiceiomimus* could probably run about 60 kilometers an hour. But heavy dinosaurs with short legs were very slow. They probably walked about four to five kilometers an hour. Slower than people walk!

For many years, people believed that dinosaurs were lazy and didn't use their brains very much. People thought they were only good at **fighting** other dinosaurs.

But now, we know much more from the study of dinosaur bones. Some dinosaur brains were quite big, so they were probably smart. And some dinosaurs lived in groups, so they didn't always fight. Scientist Jack Horner found fossils of dinosaur adults, babies, and eggs together. They lived in families, and the parents looked after the young.

And think about how long dinosaurs lived – 160 million years! That isn't bad when you think people like us have been here for only 200,000 years! Maybe dinosaurs were smarter than people think.

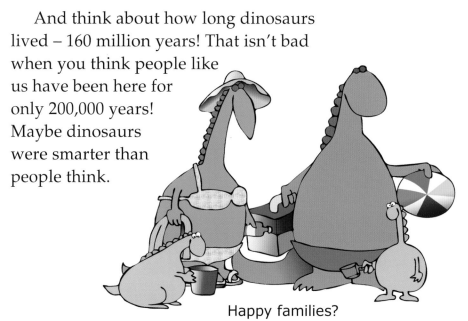

Happy families?

CHAPTER 3

Old Bones

HISTORY IS OFTEN A MYSTERY. BUT BONES CAN TELL US THE SECRETS OF THE PAST!

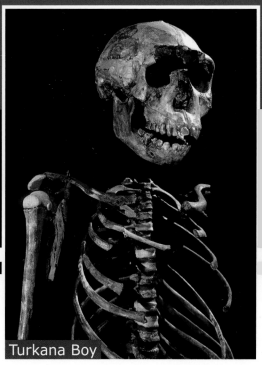

Turkana Boy

Where did humans first live? What were our ancestors[5] like?

In 1974, 40 percent of a female[6] skeleton was found in Ethiopia. Scientists called her Lucy. She lived about 3.2 million years ago. She was about 1.1 meters tall and probably weighed about 29 kilograms. Her skull was small, so she didn't have a big brain.

In 1984, another skeleton, called Turkana Boy, was found in Kenya. It's the oldest nearly complete human skeleton we have today. He lived about 1.5 million years ago. Scientists think he was between 8 and 12 years old when he died, and about 1.6 meters tall.

[5]**ancestor:** a person in your family that lived a long time ago
[6]**female:** a girl or a woman

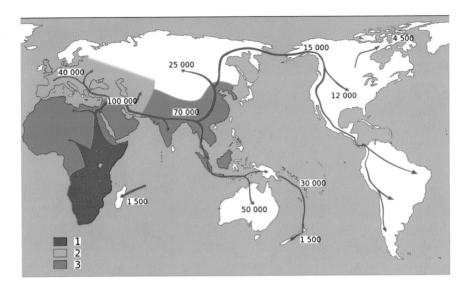

From fossils, scientists know that humans first lived in Africa. But where did they go next? Probably to Southeast Asia, but for many years scientists didn't discover any really old human bones there. Then, in 2009, a piece of skull was found in Laos. It was more than 46,000 years old and showed that early groups of people traveled through this country, maybe on their way to China.

Sometimes when we find old bones, we don't know what kind of person they came from. In 1996, a skeleton was discovered in the state of Washington, USA. Scientists called it Kennewick Man. At first, scientists said he was a white man, but Native Americans[7] said he belonged to them.

[7]**Native Americans:** the first people to live in North America

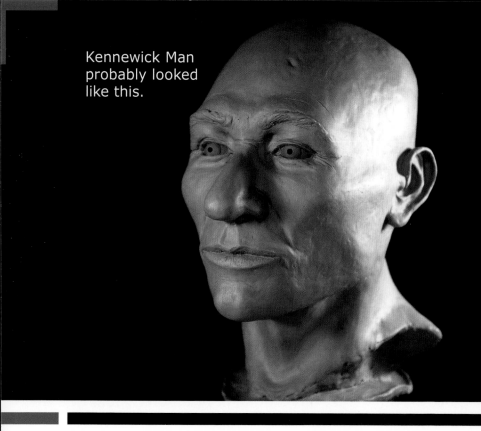

Kennewick Man probably looked like this.

The two groups started fighting over Kennewick Man. The scientists wanted to study the skeleton, but the Native Americans wanted to **bury** him. They believed this was the right thing to do. The bones were put in a museum, and the Native Americans went there often to pray.

In the end, the scientists won. They studied the skeleton and discovered Kennewick Man was about 40 years old when he died, weighed about 73 kilograms, and was 1.73 meters tall. He ate fish and other sea animals. They also discovered that he lived about 9,300 years ago! So, he wasn't white or Native American. In fact, his people probably came from southern Asia.

In 2013, Richard III, an English king who died in 1485, was suddenly in the news again. His skeleton was found under a parking lot in Leicester, England. This was exciting for science, but a problem, too. Where should they bury him? Some people said in Leicester, near where he lay. Others said London was the right place for an important king. And other people said in York, where his family was important.

And what about Columbus, the first European man to discover America, in 1492? Two cities say they have his skeleton – Seville in Spain and Santo Domingo in the Dominican Republic. First Columbus was buried in Spain, but in 1537 his bones were sent to Santo Domingo. Later, they were sent back to Spain. But people found another skeleton in Santo Domingo that they think is Colombus. So which city has the real Columbus?

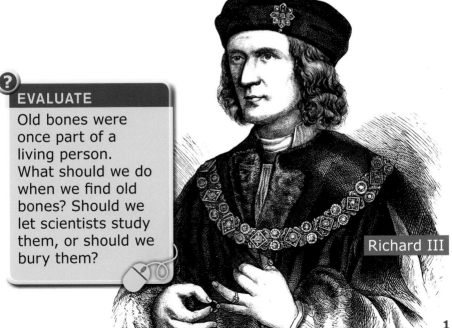

?

EVALUATE

Old bones were once part of a living person. What should we do when we find old bones? Should we let scientists study them, or should we bury them?

Richard III

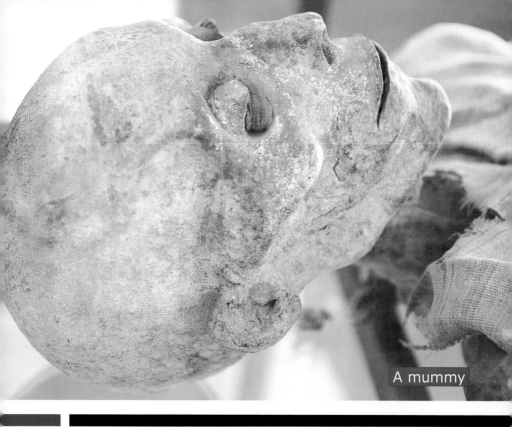

A mummy

Bones can also tell us a lot about the lives of famous people from the past. In 1922, to the surprise of the whole world, a fantastic tomb was discovered in Egypt. Inside the tomb, scientists found a lot of gold. And, of course, they found a coffin,[8] too.

Inside the coffin, there was a mummy. Long ago, when important Egyptian people died, their bodies were made into mummies. Water was taken out of the body with salt. Then special chemicals[9] were used to stop nature from destroying the body.

....

[8] **coffin:** a box we bury a dead person in
[9] **chemicals:** Scientists use these in laboratories. H_2O is the chemical name for water, for example.

18

The mummy was Tutankhamun, an important Egyptian pharaoh[10] who lived about 3,300 years ago. He became king at the age of 9 and died very young, at the age of 19. But why he died was always a mystery.

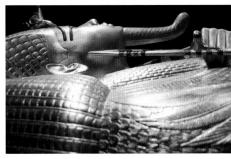
Tutankhamun's coffin

Scientists started studying Tutankhamun's mummy. In 1968, bits of bone were found in his skull. Some scientists thought maybe he died because somebody hit him on the head. Was the child king killed? Later studies showed this wasn't right. In fact, Tutankhamun wasn't a healthy boy. He had **weak** bones and a bad left foot. He probably couldn't walk very well. Maybe he died because he was sick.

More than a thousand years later, another great Egyptian pharaoh, Cleopatra, was born. In the movies Cleopatra is always a beautiful, white woman. But scientists have found the bones of Cleopatra's sister, Princess Arsinoe. Their studies show her mother was African. So maybe Cleopatra was black!

[10] **pharaoh:** the name for a king in Egypt many years ago

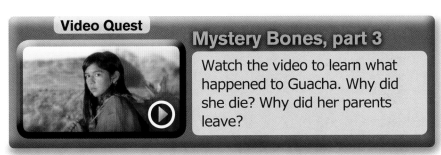

Video Quest

Mystery Bones, part 3

Watch the video to learn what happened to Guacha. Why did she die? Why did her parents leave?

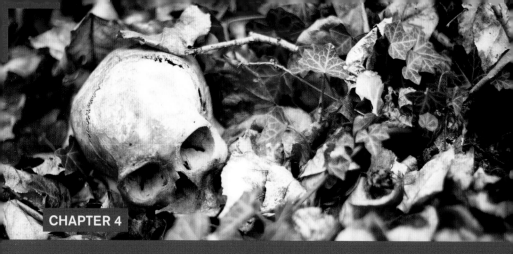

CHAPTER 4

New Bones

WHEN THERE IS A CRIME, THE POLICE HAVE TO FIND ANSWERS. SOMETIMES THEY FIND THEM BY LOOKING AT BONES!

A man is out running in the forest one morning. Suddenly, he sees something strange on the **ground**. He stops and picks it up. Then he lets it fall to the ground again. Oh no! It's a bone!

The police find more bones, but they don't have more information. Where did the bones come from? What happened? Was it an accident or a terrible **crime**?

When the police need help with these things, they contact forensic scientists – scientists who work on crimes. The scientists first decide if the bones are from a person or an animal – if there is no skull, animal bones and human bones look more or less the same.

If the bones are human, then they start to look for more information about the person.

They find out the person's age. This is easier in young bones because they are still growing. After the age of 30, people's bones are slowly destroyed, but we don't know how fast. So it's more difficult to guess the age.

The pelvis is useful in deciding if the bones belonged to a man or a woman. A woman's pelvis is usually wider but shorter than a man's.

By looking at how long the bones are, they can tell the person's height. By studying the hands, they can see if the person was right- or left-handed.

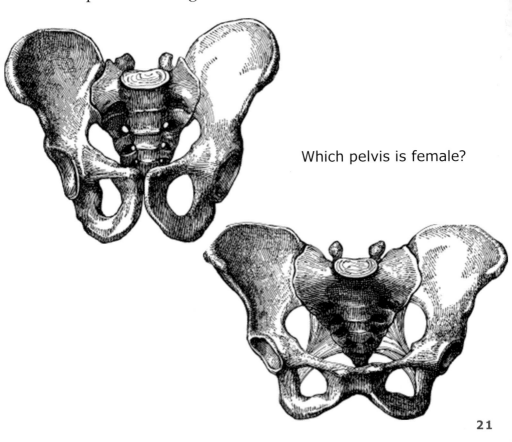

Which pelvis is female?

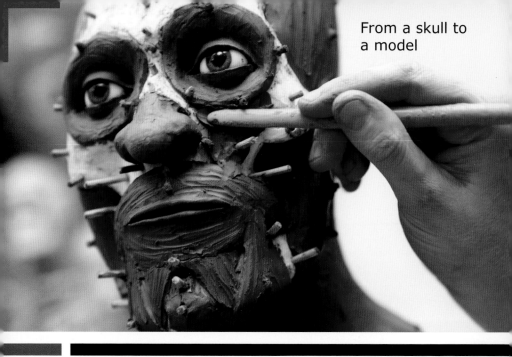

From a skull to a model

Scientists can make a model of the person's head and face from the skull. They can also put information about the skull into a computer, and a special program makes a picture of what the person probably looked like. Pictures are then put on a website about missing people.

Maybe this sounds like a horrible thing to do, but forensic scientist Erin Kimmerle says, "When the police find a skeleton, parents call from all over the country asking if it's their son or daughter. They don't rest until they know." The pictures can help these families find answers and help the police solve crimes.

?

EVALUATE

What are two good things and two bad things about the job of a forensic scientist?

Many people are interested in forensic science these days because of popular TV programs like *CSI* and *Bones*. These shows can make the job of a forensic scientist seem exciting, but is it really?

On December 28, 1978, police began digging in the garden of a house in Illinois, USA. At first, they found one bone. Forensic scientists said it was from a human arm. So they continued digging, finding bone after bone after bone.

Scientists spent many months trying to decide how many bodies there were, and which bones belonged to which body. In the end, they found the bodies of 33 young men. By studying the bones, they were able to put names to 25 of them.

The house belonged to John Wayne Gacy. Police learned that he spent years killing young men. He thought their dead bodies couldn't tell his secret. But bones talk. Gacy was executed[11] in 1994.

....

[11] **executed:** killed for doing terrible things

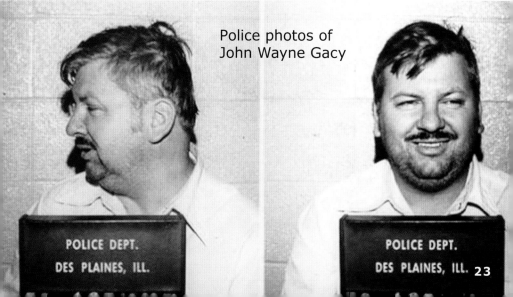

Police photos of John Wayne Gacy

POLICE DEPT.
DES PLAINES, ILL.

POLICE DEPT.
DES PLAINES, ILL.

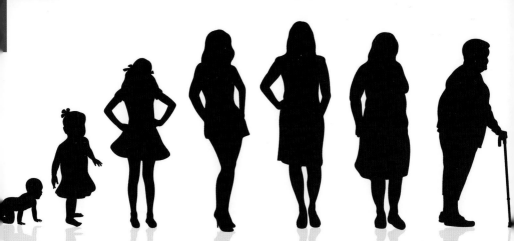

With osteoporosis, it's more difficult to stand up straight.

CHAPTER 5

What Do You Think?

WHAT ABOUT YOUR BONES? HOW HEALTHY ARE THEY?

As people grow up, they make new bone all the time. When people are older, they can have problems with their bones.

Some people get osteoporosis. This means their bones get weak, and they break easily. This happens more to women than to men, so girls and women have to be especially careful with their bones.

Read these sentences to find out how healthy your bones are. Check (✓) the ones that are true for you.

I am younger than 30.	
I am a boy or a man.	
I drink lots of milk and water.	
I don't drink a lot of coffee.	
I often eat cheese, yogurt, and green vegetables.	
I don't eat too much salt.	
I don't smoke.	
I do lots of exercise like running or walking.	
I did lots of exercise when I was a teenager.	
I spend lots of time outside in the sun.	

For every sentence that is true for you, you get one point. Add up your points, and read about your bones.

8–10 points: Congratulations! Your bones win top prize. They are strong and healthy. Keep up the good work!

5–7 points: Oh, dear! You should probably make some changes. Eat better and exercise more, or your bones will get weak!

0–4 points: Not so good. Start exercising today, and stop those bad things you're doing. Your bones need help – now!

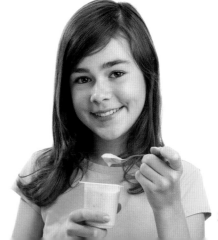

After You Read

Choose the Correct Answers

Read the sentences and choose Ⓐ, Ⓑ, Ⓒ, or Ⓓ.

1 When a child starts growing, his or her bones get _____.

Ⓐ smaller
Ⓑ harder
Ⓒ lighter
Ⓓ softer

2 Scientists can guess a person's height by looking at his or her _____.

Ⓐ femur
Ⓑ ribs
Ⓒ teeth
Ⓓ skull

3 The Chinese used dinosaur bones when somebody _____.

Ⓐ started school
Ⓑ got married
Ⓒ felt unhappy
Ⓓ was sick

4 Dinosaurs lived in this world _____.

Ⓐ for less time than humans have lived
Ⓑ a short time before humans first lived
Ⓒ much longer than humans have lived
Ⓓ at the same time as humans lived

5 Native Americans weren't happy because scientists _____.

Ⓐ wanted to bury Kennewick man
Ⓑ wanted to study Kennewick man
Ⓒ discovered Kennewick man
Ⓓ broke Kennewick man's bones

6 Tutankhamun's bones showed that he was a _____.

Ⓐ white man

Ⓑ black man

Ⓒ strong man

Ⓓ weak man

7 It's easier for forensic scientists to know the age of people who died when they were _____.

Ⓐ old

Ⓑ young

Ⓒ strong

Ⓓ weak

Complete the Text

Use the words in the box to complete the story.

bones	destroyed	mystery	secrets	skull	weighed

In 1991, two tourists were walking in the mountains between Austria and Italy when they found a man's body. Who was this **1** _____ man? Because the body was in the ice, it wasn't completely **2** _____ . When scientists studied the skeleton, they discovered its **3** _____ .

Ötzi, or Iceman, lived about 3,300 years ago. He was about 1.65 meters tall and **4** _____ about 50 kilograms. He was about 45 years old when he died. His leg **5** _____ showed that he did a lot of walking. To see what he looked like, visit the Museum of Archaeology in Bolzano, Italy. They made a model of his face from his **6** _____ .

?

APPLY

Some people make jewelry or knives from bones. Other people put bones in houses or churches. What about your family or culture? Do you do anything with bones?

Answer Key

Words to Know, page 4

1 mystery **2** skull **3** bone **4** tomb **5** fossil **6** skeleton

Words to Know, page 5

1 dig **2** secrets **3** buried **4** destroyed **5** discovering

Video Quest, page 5

It is not a normal tomb. The child was left face down in a dirty place, and there were no special things there.

Video Quest, page 9

Corn doesn't grow in the area. So maybe the child wasn't from there. Or maybe she was part of an important family who could eat special things.

Analyze, page 11   *Answers will vary.*

Evaluate, page 17   *Answers will vary.*

Video Quest, page 19

Guacha got sick and died. Her parents had to leave because they didn't want to get sick, too.

Evaluate, page 22   *Answers will vary.*

Choose the Correct Answers, page 26

1 B **2** A **3** D **4** C **5** B **6** D **7** B

Complete the Text, page 27

1 mystery **2** destroyed **3** secrets **4** weighed **5** bones **6** skull

Apply, page 27   *Answers will vary.*